MW00988605

Cancer and The Lord's Prayer

Hope & Healing Through History's Greatest Prayer

by Greg Anderson

Copyright ©2006 by Greg Anderson.

All rights reserved. No part of this book may be reproduced in any form without written permission from the publisher.

Meredith Books
1716 Locust Street
Des Moines, Iowa 50309–3023
meredithbooks.com

Printed in the United States of America.
First Edition.
Library of Congress Control Number: 2006921519
ISBN-10: 0-696-23256-1
ISBN-13: 978-0-696-23256-5

Jordan House™ and the Jordan House logo are trademarks of Meredith Corporation.

The ideas and suggestions contained in this book are not intended as a substitute for consulting with your physician. All matters regarding your health require medical supervision.

Table of Contents

Acknowledgments

To cancer patients everywhere—there is hope! Tap into the power of prayer. Transform your moments of fear and hopelessness into a life filled with faith and hope and love. It's here. Open your heart.

I am an exceedingly blessed person. One of my greatest blessings is my dear wife, Linda—thank you for your unconditional love and support. I am so grateful that God brought us together.

Preface: Author's Invitation

Dear Reader,

I want to teach you to pray a very familiar prayer in a new and daring way. It's the Lord's Prayer taught by Jesus and recorded in the Bible.

I first learned this prayer as a very young child. It's always been part of my life. I repeated it every week in Sunday school and in church. Sadly it became mere ritual.

Years later I was diagnosed with cancer and given 30 days to live. The Greatest Prayer took on new and vital meaning, and it became the basis of my healing. Today it is the spiritual foundation of my entire life.

Will you join me for an up close and personal exploration of the Lord's Prayer?

I hope you will not only join me in praying this prayer but also in living it.

Greg Anderson

The Lord's Prayer

Our Father which art in heaven,
Hallowed be thy name.
Thy kingdom come.
Thy will be done in earth,
as it is in heaven.
Give us this day our daily bread.
And forgive us our debts,
as we forgive our debtors.
And lead us not into temptation,
but deliver us from evil:
For thine is the kingdom, and the power,
and the glory, for ever.

chapter

1

The Greatest Prayer

The little book you are holding is about what happens when ordinary Christians who are going through cancer decide to no longer settle for the rituals of their faith and instead reach out—and actually live out—the very real promises of Jesus. In fact, that is exactly the type of spiritual journey that God honors with many different kinds of healings, sometimes even cures.

My journey of substituting a living faith for empty and tired ritual began in the tiny spare bedroom of a small ranch house in Southern California. I was put there, I thought, to be out of the way, not to bother anyone. I was put there to die.

It was mid-1984 when I began to cough. The cough simply would not stop. I went to a doctor who ordered a battery of medical tests. It was soon discovered I had lung cancer. I agreed to surgery and my left lung was removed. I thought my troubles were behind me.

Four months later I was back in the same hospital with the same surgeon. This time I had a lump at the base of my neck. The cancer had spread throughout my lymph system. The surgeon opened and then closed. The cancer was too advanced. There was nothing more to do.

The next day he came into my hospital room and uttered words I will never forget. In a quiet tone of voice he said, "Greg, I don't know how to tell you this, but the tiger is out of the cage. Your cancer has come roaring back. I would give you about 30 days to live." That was December 1984. I moved back home.

I prayed. My wife prayed. People at our church prayed. Actually prayer had been part of my life ever since I could remember. In the home of my youth, our family prayed at meals, before bed, and, of course, on Sunday morning. Linda, my wife, and I had done the same in our family.

Following the diagnosis of cancer, I prayed more fervently. In the middle of the night, alone in that tiny bedroom, I pleaded with God to keep me from death. I believed intensified prayer was the answer, the key that would unlock health and healing.

But even those times of prayerful fervor failed to establish a constant and ever-deepening intimacy with God.

I continued to deteriorate physically. At one point I was down to 112 pounds. My skin was ashen gray, and I was on morphine to ease the pain.

I clearly recall looking down at my thin wrists with their many tendons and bones sticking out, thinking "Well, it's probably true. I guess I am going to die."

Those moments of self-pity plunged me into despair and hopelessness. Fear crowded out my faith. The downward spiral engulfed me.

Not knowing what to say or do, I instinctively prayed, without being mindful of the prayer's meaning, "Our Father, which art in heaven …." End of prayer. End of ritual.

"Lord, I really want to live," I'd pray. Sometimes in the middle of the night, I walked out back to sit on our patio. In the dark of night I would speak, "Lord, what exactly can I do?" I wondered about God's silence. In some of those lonely moments, I seriously questioned the existence of God and wondered about the depth and power of my faith.

Maybe it was the silence that kept me turning back to what I knew from my earliest recollections. I simply continued to pray, "Our Father which art in heaven, Hallowed be thy name …."

Something in this prayer instinctively touched me, even though I did not actually understand all that much about it. Yes, I vaguely remembered that this was the model prayer Jesus taught his disciples. And yes, I knew it was somewhere in the Bible, but I didn't even know the chapter and verse.

Early one morning, I prayed the Lord's Prayer again. But that morning, my spirit was eager to learn more about it. I determined I would find it in the Scriptures.

I pulled up a chair to our kitchen table, picked up my Bible and thought, "OK, if Jesus taught this, it must be in the Gospels, either Matthew, Mark, Luke, or John." So I opened to Matthew and started reading. I was determined to understand more.

I didn't have to read far. There, in the sixth chapter

of Matthew, the prayer first appears. I pored over those verses again and again. I searched with all my mind and spirit for the answers God might have for a frightened, confused person such as myself.

The next morning, I prayed the prayer again, this time just as it was written.

And the next morning.

And the next.

More than 20 years later, I continue.

This single prayer has been the central point of power in my recovery from an almost-certain cancer death sentence.

Now, in the pages of this book, I want to introduce you to the amazing power and truth found in the Lord's Prayer. I want to prepare you to expect the hope and healing held within its promises. And I want to encourage you to make this prayer a regular, meaningful, vital part of your life.

Why do I think this discipline will change your health and your life? It's because of my experience and the similar experiences of hundreds of other cancer survivors around the world with whom I've shared these principles. It's because the intelligent, mindful application of the Lord's Prayer absolutely changes lives.

The greatest prayer

While some things in life are just not important, others are clearly important. Still other things are absolutely critical. The Lord's Prayer definitely falls into the third category.

Think of it. This prayer stands across the entire spectrum of Christian expression as the most important of all. It was first spoken by Jesus, is the best known of his teachings, and is the most often quoted. If there is just one common denominator in all Christianity, this is it.

You'll find the Lord's Prayer in Matthew and in Luke. It follows Jesus' teachings of the Beatitudes, his admonition to turn the other cheek, and his instructions on giving to the needy. Jesus then turns to the most important subject of all: how to pray.

I have discussed this with hundreds of lifelong Christians who, like me, have recited this prayer thousands of times. Jesus warned of praying in vain repetitions, and that was certainly my experience with this prayer. But then, as I thought through its message, I saw this prayer come to life. Hundreds of people have shared similar experiences.

The Lord's Prayer is the essential recipe for healing the soul. I believe Jesus authored it for the specific purpose of our personal spiritual growth so that those who make it a central part of their lives, those who pray it regularly and pray it with deepening understanding, will be rewarded with a healing of the spirit.

The Bible refers to this as being "born again." Born again means the spirit of Jesus Christ takes center stage in your heart, and you become a new, or a renewed, person. It is the change of spirit that matters.

Mere intellectual acquisition of knowledge does not change the soul. At best, that results in rituals with some good works thrown in for good measure. The Lord's Prayer is designed to bring about the soul change that generates new people, new health, and new life.

I marvel at the structural beauty of the Lord's Prayer. It's awe-inspiring to understand the spiritual progression Jesus was teaching. And best of all, the prayer meets every person's need at his or her level of spiritual understanding.

For mature Christians, the prayer offers a powerful way of life. It opens the way for God's amazing truths, blessings, and favor as a daily part of life—a life that experiences the miracles of God, a life lived in the presence of God.

For people who are ready for rapid spiritual growth, the prayer is perfect. It offers a gateway for thinking about and being alert for signs and directions from God wherever they go, with whomever they meet, and whatever the circumstances. Try it. I know you will begin to see God in people and places you never before realized.

If you are a spiritual child, the Lord's Prayer is the road map, your direction for travel. It's true; right here in this prayer you will find your way. Keep mining the prayer's meaning and direction. You will reap many rewards.

I believe Jesus also constructed this prayer to be "theology proof." The spiritual message of the Lord's Prayer is simple, direct, uncomplicated, and accessible. Jesus did not erect any doctrinal barriers between God and humanity. The prayer carries the whole message of Christianity within it, no manmade additions necessary.

Dare to believe it. The Greatest Prayer is all about living the great life—now! It's for you. It's for me. It's especially for people with cancer.

Prayer treatment

Cancer can open many doors. One of the most important is the door to your heart. When was the last time you fully opened your heart to God? When was the most recent healing—physical, emotional, or spiritual— you personally experienced? If you're like most believers I have talked to, it's been a long time, if ever. In fact you might even be uncertain if you are able to have that kind of experience, or even if you should ask for it.

What I have to share with you is a totally new perspective on health and healing. At one of our Cancer:

Spirit-Mind-Body Retreats in Baltimore, I shared about the healing power of the Lord's Prayer. After dinner that evening, a woman said, "I started praying this prayer the hour after my diagnosis. I haven't stopped. That was eight years ago. I am cancer free."

Another participant agreed. He said he had been carefully, mindfully saying the Lord's Prayer for the last two years. His life and health had never been better.

For 20 years I have personally prayed this prayer. Today my life is literally one miracle after another. And since 1989, my medical records have stated, "This patient is clinically free of any signs of cancer."

Wherever I go to share this message, countless numbers of people speak of the mighty hope and healing found in the Greatest Prayer of all.

I wish the same for you. Because you are reading this book, I believe you share my desire to live life to the fullest—physically, emotionally, and spiritually. You want a miracle from God so you can be a miracle for God. It's not that you want anything less for others, but you want to live life fully blessed by God, no matter what medical science might have to say.

Believe it. God has miracles in store for you. But you have a part to play in attaining them. I know that may sound impossible. It may even seem suspicious, a claim without merit, a promise that could be manipulated.

It is really quite simple; God, our Father, seeks your spiritual transformation. And with a few commitments, all found in the Lord's Prayer, you can proceed through your cancer journey with the confidence and expectation that your Heavenly Father will be with you—no matter what.

Or you might wish to consider it this way: Instead of fearfully, grudgingly going through with your next cancer treatment, do something unthinkable. Take this Greatest Prayer with you every moment. Pray over your cancer treatment and all the people associated with its delivery. And keep praying this prayer, thoughtfully and reverently, through treatment, after treatment, and every day of your recovery.

At the very moment you begin this discipline, a new treatment is put in place. It's prayer treatment. It becomes central, the most important of all your treatments. All other treatments, including surgery, radiation, and chemotherapy, become complementary to your mainstream healing strategy—your Lord's Prayer protocol.

When you make this commitment, you enter into the great currents of God's grace. God's power will surround you. He will give you peace. God will give you abundant life. He may even cure your cancer.

If all this is what you desire, read on.

chapter

2

Our Father which art in heaven,
Hallowed be thy name.
Thy kingdom come.
Thy will be done in earth,
as it is in heaven.
Give us this day our daily bread.
And forgive us our debts,
as we forgive our debtors.
And lead us not into temptation,
but deliver us from evil:
For thine is the kingdom, and the power,
and the glory, for ever.

*Y*ou're in the waiting room outside the surgical suites of a busy hospital. Perhaps 15 people are sharing the waiting room with you. You're there because your spouse is going through an operation. The others are there for family and friends who are also either in surgery or waiting to hear a physician's report.

A doctor appears and sits next to a woman just across from you. The report is not good. The surgeon was able to remove only a small part of the husband's tumor. More treatment will certainly be required. The future is uncertain.

As the doctor leaves, the exhausted spouse is looking particularly grim. She breaks down and begins to weep.

Without thinking, someone slips over and sits down beside her, holds her hand, and begins reciting the Lord's Prayer.

Before you know it, three or four others in that waiting room have joined in.

You don't know these people, not a name or even a home town. But you respond and join in that prayer. Soon everyone in the room is saying the same prayer.

The Lord's Prayer and a moment of crisis are the only things you all have in common, but it is enough. You form a bond of fellowship based on that prayer in that extremely difficult moment.

A constant prayer

Is it possible that God wants you to be immersed in that same prayer on a daily and hourly basis? I've met so many well-meaning and devoted Christians who dismiss the power of the Lord's Prayer saying, "It's too formal" or "I feel like it is meant to be reserved for church."

Maybe you think that too. If you do, I want to help you understand that the Lord's Prayer is not just a formal statement of ritual reserved for special occasions. No, it is exactly the kind of prayer our Father wants to hear. It clearly points out the path to healing.

When the disciples asked Jesus to teach them to pray, he taught them this Greatest Prayer and all its components: praising and acknowledging God's holiness, petitioning God for his presence and daily supply, and requesting forgiveness, guidance, and deliverance.

It all starts with the simple words "Our Father." Simple? Yes. But not simplistic.

This doesn't sound like the start of a life-changing prayer, does it?

"Our Father." Oh, what a statement! For the cancer patient, those two words are not only a complete statement of correct theological understanding, but they are also healing; they are life!

Those words summarize the nature of God and the nature of humankind. That phrase tells us all we need to know about three people: God, myself, and my neighbor. Those two words form the basis of the journey through cancer.

"Our Father." Jesus gave us this clear and uncomplicated statement as our starting point. It establishes that the relationship between God and you and me is that of father and child.

What comes to your mind when you say, "Our Father"? Many people, myself included, have experienced difficult, dysfunctional, even abusive relationships with their earthly fathers. And many others have fathers who were physically absent or emotionally unreachable. Saying "Our Father" may bring thoughts of irritation, mistrust, abandonment, or much worse.

Thankfully we have another father, a totally loving Heavenly Father. It is to this relationship the Lord's Prayer guides us.

As I started to examine the Lord's Prayer in greater and greater depth, as I continued to talk to other cancer patients and family members about its meaning, a pattern became clear. When the "Our Father" is commenced, an experience of ritual begins to unfold.

A prayer beyond ritual

Certainly there are good things to be found in ritual. Comfort, for one. A sense of the known brings with it a certain hope, an easing of grief or uncertainty.

And consolation. A long-established ceremonial action brings with it a sense of permanency that all is well in this world, perhaps even with a diagnosis of cancer. Ritual has its place.

But healing and victory are found when you and I take the "Our Father" promises way beyond the bounds of ritual. We're talking nothing short of transformation, the living out of a new life—mentally, emotionally, and spiritually.

Yes, I appreciate the many levels of understanding of the Lord's Prayer. Clearly there is a social component that meets people at the point of needing to belong, of needing human as well as divine support. And comfort in community brought by ritual is obviously found in the Greatest Prayer. But neither ritual nor comfort heals.

By far the least understood dimension of the Lord's Prayer is its transforming power. God is constantly trying to plant new seeds of spiritual potential in you and me. He's trying to increase and expand our faith and our vision of what is possible.

God wants to take us to new levels of victory, to deeper levels of spiritual understanding, and to higher levels of life experience. "Our Father" defines our roles in this transformation.

God is our Father. We are his children. Jesus says it's all about parent and child. The relationship is settled.

Elsewhere, throughout Scripture, that relationship is further defined. God is our loving parent. He wants only what's best for us. God is not some relentless, cruel despot, a tyrant who punishes.

In Matthew 7, we receive the exceedingly good news, "If you, then, though you are evil, know how to give good gifts to your children, how much more will your Father in heaven give good gifts to those who ask him!"

God is the perfect parent dealing with his sometimes, many times, imperfect children.

And there's more good news. If God is our Father, we are his offspring. That is very good news indeed. As offspring, we are without doubt similar to and made in the image of our parent. Just as our Father is loving spirit, we must be essentially loving spirits also, even though appearances may indicate otherwise.

Dear friend, meditate upon this relationship. Continue to meditate often until you have gained a true understanding of what this relationship really means. God is the real, eternal, all-powerful, omnipresent, and loving Father of humankind. You have nothing to fear, not even cancer.

Be happy. You are safe. You are loved.

"Our Father." Jesus placed this statement first. It

is the Greatest Prayer's vivid reminder that God is our loving Father and that all is well, very well indeed. Our realization and acknowledgment of this relationship form the required starting point of our transformation; they are the seeds of our healing.

Challenges to victory

I believe there are very real forces that do not wish these seeds to bear fruit in you. Call them negative thinking, the enemy, or the devil. By any name, helplessness and despair set out to uproot the seeds of hope and healing God planted. In order to allow that seed to grow, you and I must remain focused on "Our Father" and all those two words imply.

Constantly meditate on this relationship and live a life that is pleasing and honorable. Thank God for his faithfulness no matter what the doctor's report might say. And before long, you'll begin to see healing on all levels and blessings of every kind. You will experience a transformed life.

Finally, draw strength from others. Note that Jesus said it is "Our" Father, not "My" Father. He is teaching us the truth that we are all children of one father. Yes, all of us. It's the brotherhood of humankind right in the Greatest Prayer.

"Our Father" implies that we strive for peace and

goodwill toward all, that we acknowledge we are our brothers' keepers, and that we are to pray not only for ourselves but for everyone.

"Our Father." Much power is contained in those simple, innocent-looking words. It's transforming. It's healing. It's real.

I pray you will discover this power for yourself. In Romans 8:16–17 we are given the assurance that "we are children of God, and if children, then heirs—heirs of God and joint heirs with Christ." So I implore you to stop saying "Our Father" on Sunday, only to spend the rest of the week living like an orphan. Act on the belief we hold so dear. Since God is our Father, we simply need not wander through life-threatening illness like some lost and powerless waif.

Through these simple words, through this Greatest Prayer, you can change your health and your life.

So why not start? Why not now?

"Our Father …."

chapter

3

Our Father *which art in heaven,*
Hallowed be thy name.
Thy kingdom come.
Thy will be done in earth,
as it is in heaven.
Give us this day our daily bread.
And forgive us our debts,
as we forgive our debtors.
And lead us not into temptation,
but deliver us from evil:
For thine is the kingdom, and the power,
and the glory, for ever.

The relationship is established. God is the parent and we are the children. Now Jesus teaches us more about God's nature and our role.

Setting aside ritual and reaching for new health and new life require us to develop a constant and ever-deepening intimacy with God. We are now shown how.

Practicing the presence of God

Brother Lawrence is one of history's great spiritual masters. Born Nicholas Herman in the Lorraine province, France, around 1605, he came from a humble background and was an unlearned man. He was converted to Christianity in 1629 and, after being a soldier and a footman, entered the religious community of the Carmelites in Paris. It was there, as a lay brother, that he took the name of Brother Lawrence. He remained with the Carmelites until his death in 1691.

In the community he worked most of the time as a helper in the kitchen. In these humble surroundings he became known for his simple, practical, and powerful faith. In all circumstances and at all times throughout his life, he practiced a constant connection with God.

During his lifetime, Brother Lawrence's influence spread throughout France. After his death his writings, primarily letters, were edited and printed in two volumes.

In these writings we discover a very inspiring way of life consisting of a simple and constant practice of awareness of the presence of God. This he maintained by meditating unceasingly on God with high thoughts.

Brother Lawrence teaches us that amid our outward affairs and daily preoccupations, it is possible to cultivate a life of contemplation. Every Christian has the ability, through the grace of God, to enjoy an ongoing, deeply intimate fellowship with his Creator wherever he is, whatever he is doing, and in any and all circumstances, even struggling with cancer.

"The time of business [he wrote] does not with me differ from the time of prayer; and in the clatter of my kitchen, while several persons are at the same time calling for different things, I possess God in as great a tranquillity as if I were upon my knees at the blessed sacrament."

In the truest sense, our lives can also be a constant prayer. Brother Lawrence gives us a model of holy delight, evidence that a spiritual focus changes everything. At the very least, his life teaches that living prayerfully is much more than pausing to talk to God for a few minutes on Sunday morning.

Enlarging God's nature

That is what Jesus is describing and implying when he says our Father is "in heaven" in the second phrase of the Greatest Prayer. Having shown us that God and humankind are parent and child respectively, he now enlarges God's nature and describes our responsibilities.

Jesus teaches that God is in heaven and humankind is here on earth. God, always loving and caring, is constantly seeking connection with us. God is trying to bring heaven on earth to us and through us. Our task is to connect, to be like Brother Lawrence and practice the presence of God.

Our highest destiny is to be an expression of God in all manner of glorious and wonderful ways. We have been given the journey of cancer, in part, as an opportunity for that expression. As we are one with God, but not one and the same, we show his heavenly love to all we meet on this surprising portion of our earthly journey.

The practice and expression of this God presence is one of the most profound manners of healing.

We develop this practice and expression by consistently thinking about God and being alert for signs of God wherever we go. By paying prayerful attention every waking hour, we are less likely to rush past the healing opportunities that are constantly being presented in our lives.

I want you to begin to believe that God is always trying to speak to you and through you. Become constantly watchful in the experiences, the people, the scripture, and the communication that comes your way. Much of it may need to be filtered through God's Word. But if we are truly living in the presence of God, we can then be ready to receive and act on instructions from our heavenly Father.

Opportunities to pray

Being in this state of constant readiness may sound very difficult. But it is actually quite simple to constantly see life through spiritual eyes.

Brother Lawrence saw an opportunity to pray as the potatoes were peeled. You and I can pray while waiting in line at the supermarket or whenever we are stopped at a red light or wherever we find ourselves.

While I lay on the table of the linear accelerator and the radiation therapy was administered, I silently prayed, "Lord, use this treatment to heal me. I welcome your healing touch through these beams of light and energy. I am yours. Use me for your greater purposes. Amen and amen."

Pray everywhere. You will open your life to an endless stream of God-given opportunity. This is connection, and it requires two-way prayer:

> We speak.
> God listens.
> God speaks.
> We listen.

Our willingness to listen is the most important part. If we train ourselves to listen for God's voice, we will hear it.

Listen carefully. Healing speaks softly. Most of the time it whispers. But if we just still ourselves and listen, we will sense the direction of God.

Your Father in heaven is trying to make his presence known in and through you, even through the cancer journey.

Listen. Your Heavenly Father is trying to reach you.

Listen. Cultivate an ever-increasing, deeply intimate practice of the presence of God.

Listen. It's a sure way of bringing a little more heaven here on earth.

Listen. You will find your healing!

Listen.

chapter

4

Our Father which art in heaven,

Hallowed be thy name,

Thy kingdom come.

Thy will be done in earth,

as it is in heaven.

Give us this day our daily bread.

And forgive us our debts,

as we forgive our debtors.

And lead us not into temptation,

but deliver us from evil:

For thine is the kingdom, and the power,

and the glory, for ever.

*S*hakespeare asked, "What's in a name?" In the Bible, the name of something or someone defined its essential character, its nature. A man and his name were so intimately connected that "to kill the name" of an individual amounted to the same thing as murdering him. His name defined his future.

I feel the same dynamic is sometimes at work today. I have an acquaintance whose given name is actually "Stormy." His life has been one storm after another, including an arrest and jail time for selling drugs. His latest storm is cancer.

Jesus called the name of God "hallowed." For cancer patients, that is very good news indeed. Although "hallowed" has several meanings, including holy and sacred, it is actually derived from the Greek word "healed."

Our entire interpretation of the Lord's Prayer could be viewed in a radically different way:

> Our Father in heaven,
> Healing be your name.

When I understood the origin of "hallowed," I started to pray the Greatest Prayer slightly differently:

> Our Father in heaven,
> Hallowed and healing be your name.

By explicitly stating the dimension of healing in the Greatest Prayer, the full intent, the whole and deeper meaning of "hallowed" comes more vividly to life. "Healing" does not take away from the Lord's Prayer but simply makes its meaning clearer.

Place for prayer

For the patient going through cancer, this clarity is important. Our awareness of the nature of God, especially as defined by the name of God, and our choices in our relationship to God are entirely under our control. And it is ultimately our mindfulness of and attunement to God that determine our well-being, even our physical health.

For more than 20 years, I have studied why people get well. Medicine has its place, to be sure. But it probably plays a lesser role than most people give it.

Just as important are positive attitudes, self-awareness, self-motivation, healthy diet, and consistent exercise. And above all, our spiritual connection makes a huge difference in the outcome of the cancer experience.

In fact, if I had to prescribe one and only one cancer treatment for every patient, it would not be surgery, radiation, or chemotherapy. Once again, these techniques certainly do have a place. But if limited to just one treatment, my choice would be prayer therapy.

Besides the obvious spiritual benefit, numerous clinical trials show evidence of the healing power in prayer. It is the way to connect to our God, who possesses unlimited healing resources. Those resources await our claim, and the Greatest Prayer reveals them.

To unlock healing, you need to believe something with complete sincerity. I have come to understand that our beliefs about God's hallowed nature are central to what we need to believe to experience healing. Compare the following characteristics of human nature and divine nature:

Human nature	Divine nature
Pessimism	Optimism
Pride	Wisdom
Intolerance	Acceptance
Cruelty	Benevolence
Selfishness	Selflessness
Self-pity	Compassion
Sadness	Joy
Guilt	Forgiveness
Fear	Faith
Despair	Hope
Anger, hatred	Love, goodwill
Dis-ease	Peace

There are many more characteristics, but this much we know to be scientifically true: The characteristics of human nature are all stressful and involve negative responses. These include the activation of our sympathetic nervous system, increased production of adrenaline and cortisol, loss of magnesium, physical exhaustion, and impaired immune function.

The characteristics of divine nature are restorative. Our autonomic nervous system responds and we physically and emotionally experience greater equilibrium and well-being.

That, I believe, is what Jesus was teaching us when he admonished us to pray, "Hallowed [healing] be thy name." The fact is God is not merely worthy of our awe and worship, but he is complete and perfect and altogether good, even if we might not realize it given our current health circumstances.

Awareness of God

Remember, your awareness of God and your relationship with God are entirely under your control. Stop thinking that God sent cancer as a punishment for your imperfect ways. That is simply not God's nature. Even worse, by thinking and believing that way, you are giving power to your illness, making it even more difficult to conquer.

Start thinking about God as healer, the Almighty, the Good Shepherd, your Redeemer, and your Savior. Live out the promise of Romans 8:28 that ". . . all things work together for good to them that love God, to them who are called according to his purpose." It's true. God can take any situation, even your cancer, and use it in a way that brings blessings to you and countless others.

How you think about God, what you believe God can do in your life, and what God can do in and through your illness really do matter a great deal. Believe it. No matter where you are right now in your cancer journey, God has great good in store for you.

Begin to think the way God thinks. Break out of the pessimism, self-pity, fear, and despair. Think optimism, joy, faith, hope, and love. Thank God for all the blessings he is giving to you. Pray that God will use you and this illness for good.

When you do, God will clearly show up in many unexpected ways to perform many types of healing.

What's in a name? It's healing:

> Our Father which art in heaven,
> Healing be thy name.

chapter
5

Our Father which art in heaven,
Hallowed be thy name.

Thy kingdom come.
Thy will be done in earth,
as it is in heaven.

Give us this day our daily bread.
And forgive us our debts,
as we forgive our debtors.
And lead us not into temptation,
but deliver us from evil:
For thine is the kingdom, and the power,
and the glory, for ever.

OK, you've shared some of these ideas with the people closest to you. You said that listening for your Heavenly Father and understanding God's true nature will lead you to better embrace this powerful force called "healing." And your family and friends looked at you like you were slightly deranged. In fact, one of them said something like, "Are you nuts?"

Your well-meaning brother-in-law heard about your new quest and called to talk you into trying the new experimental cancer therapy he just heard about on the evening news.

Sometimes it's disheartening. Having dared to believe there was more to cancer than cells gone awry and increasingly toxic, invasive, and experimental cancer treatments, you've now been the recipient of a bucketful of cold water courtesy of some of your closest family and friends. Suddenly your newfound hope seems all wet.

Sound familiar? Maybe your old doubts threaten to squash your burgeoning faith. Maybe a recent medical test seems to confirm that cancer really is just cell biology gone haywire. After all, who can prove there is actually a biology of faith and hope? And besides, people with years of medical training keep saying the only treatment is more medical treatment. They're the experts. Aren't they to be believed?

Face it. You're in a quandary. You have embraced God's healing promises as your own, resolved to live in the constant presence of your Heavenly Father, but now your medical team and much of your entire support network are questioning your good sense.

When many cancer patients find themselves in this kind of paradox—torn between hope and hopelessness— they often feel afraid, misled, and abandoned. Those were certainly my feelings.

Brought to your knees

Four months after I had my lung removed, I was back in the same hospital with the same surgeon. He would now operate on the grapefruit-size lump protruding from the base of my neck. He opened but then he closed, unwilling and unable to remove the cancer without leaving me severely incapacitated. The next day he delivered his 30-days-to-live prognosis.

The news was devastating. I felt betrayed. Had my fervent prayers been completely ignored? What sort of cruelty was this? Angrily I asked, "God, do you even exist? Where are you?" It was my lowest point, my darkest hour.

Cancer brought me physically, emotionally, and spiritually to my knees. And given all the miracles I have experienced since then, I have decided that is a pretty good place to stay.

It also brought me back to the Lord's Prayer and to those startling clauses, "Thy kingdom come, thy will be done." Could it possibly be that this was all God's will for my life? From where I was, it sure didn't look like it.

Your kingdom come. Your will be done.

I recalled a lecture by Rick Warren I had heard about a year earlier. He taught his interpretation of those words, and the one point I took away from that message was we are to be ever occupied in helping bring heaven to earth. That was a surprising idea to me then, and it was a surprising idea to me now, especially at this hour when I was facing what seemed like my imminent death.

But there it was, this challenging clause, right in the middle of the Greatest Prayer, the very prayer taught by Jesus. "Thy kingdom come. Thy will be done in earth, as it is in heaven."

Wow! What if I allowed that this statement was literally true and that it applied directly to my life, even when I had just been given 30 days to live? At the very least, I needed to explore this possibility.

Why on earth are we here?

It's not all about you and me. Our temporary assignments on this planet at this hour are, ultimately, all about God. He is the reason everything exists, including you and me. And we exist to express God's glory.

Especially for those of us who profess the Christian walk, it is our God-appointed duty to help establish the Kingdom of God here on earth. Another way of saying this is that our job is to bring more and more of God's plans and ideas into reality here and now.

Your Kingdom, Lord. Your will, Lord. As you want, Lord. Here, Lord. In my life, Lord. Now, Lord. That is exactly why we are here.

For the person diagnosed with cancer, this can seem like a very frightening proposition. In fact, it's asking a great deal.

We are attached to life, to living. Praying "Thy will be done" means we may have to give up living as we know it. It may mean we give up our life here on earth. This has scary elements, even for people of deepest faith.

This whole shift requires us to set aside our preferences and demands and substitute God's in their place. This is a simple intellectual exercise for many theologians. But for the person who is battling a life-threatening illness, this is downright difficult. That's because most of us believe we know what's best for ourselves. Even more, we believe we can tell God exactly what to do to fulfill our desires.

That's why praying "Thy will be done" is so frightening. When it's cancer, we find it very common for patients to pray, "Heal me." Even the most spiritual among us may pray, "Yes, Lord, your will be done. But by the way, could that will please be to remove all of this cancer from my body?" Our personal wishes always seem to get in the way of the unconditional acceptance of God's will.

One of the most powerful reasons to pray "Thy kingdom come, thy will be done" is that our knowledge is so limited. As cancer patients, we assume that perfect health in a short period of time is the best thing for us. But is that really what's best?

In my own experience, upon diagnosis, I immediately prayed for healing. It was not to be. The cancer came back. However, if I had not had the recurrence and been told I had 30 days to live, I do not believe I would have surrendered my life to the will of God. If I had not surrendered, I very much doubt that I would have started an international cancer outreach that today brings help and hope to more than 5 million people in five different countries each year.

Illness is not judgment

Your will be done. This does not encourage a step back in time. For a very long span of human history, illness and death were believed to occur when one lost favor with God. This sentiment survives in different forms today. But I do not believe illness is God's judgment, even though he might use illness for his higher purpose.

Higher purpose. That's what God is seeking to do with your cancer experience. Your business is to help bring a little bit of heaven here on earth. Too often we think narrowly, selfishly seeking only that our will be done. We try to set up our own agenda, putting in place our own plans instead of being about our heavenly Father's business.

Virtually all our dis-ease arises out of this conflict of trying to work apart from God. It may even be the spiritual root of our cancer.

But life is not about us. We must always make plans and live our life with reference and deference to God. We can be neither successful nor happy nor well if we are seeking any other end than "thy will be done."

Whatever our desire may be, whether it is for our health, our wealth, or our relationships, if we seek to serve ourselves first instead of God, we are only placing an order for trouble, disappointment, dis-ease, and unhappiness.

Pause from your reading for just a moment to open your mind and spirit to these next few words: Cancer has spiritual significance.

God intends to use this experience for good, even if evil seems to be winning out at the moment. Romans

8:28, a verse I've quoted previously, explains this truth: "And we know that all things work together for good to them that love God, to them who are called according to his purpose." Note that the verse doesn't say "God will always work things out the way I want." Obviously that is not the case. Nor does it say "God always creates happy endings here on earth." By human standards, there are many unhappy endings on earth.

When we pray "Thy will be done," we are anchoring our eternal hope in the promises of Christ. This is not just some positive thinking with a gloss of prayer. It is an acknowledgment that God is in complete control of our lives and that he loves us. We are part of his divine plan, and even our experience of cancer has a place in this plan.

And where does it all lead? For us to become more Christ-like. That is cancer's spiritual gift. To love God more, to be called to living our lives on purpose for him, no matter how long we have been given.

Your kingdom, Lord. Your will, Lord. Here, Lord. Now, Lord.

That's healing.

chapter
6

Our Father which art in heaven,
Hallowed be thy name.
Thy kingdom come.
Thy will be done in earth,
as it is in heaven.

Give us this day our daily bread.

And forgive us our debts,
as we forgive our debtors.
And lead us not into temptation,
but deliver us from evil:
For thine is the kingdom, and the power,
and the glory, for ever.

J recently participated in a 10K hike it/bike it/walk/run. It was to benefit a local charity that established and maintains a walking trail in our community. This was a first for me, and considering I now have only one lung, I didn't know quite what to expect.

The day was hot, and shortly after the start, I became concerned about dehydration. But at the second kilometer marker I was pleasantly surprised to find a provisions station. Here, under a tent, race organizers had everything: water, juice, fresh oranges, even a nurse with bandages just in case some walker or runner raised a blister. There were even a couple of portable toilets too.

The race organizers had it all under control. An identical station was placed every two kilometers, and a veritable village of provisions awaited us just past the finish line. We were provided for in every way.

So, too, it is in our lives. Because we are children of a loving heavenly father, we can expect God to provide for everything we need. Please recognize that this is about need as determined by God, not want as determined by you or me.

"Give us this day our daily bread." When Jesus taught this portion of the Lord's Prayer, I believe he was thinking of much more than bread. Clearly he included food, clothing, and shelter under the meaning of bread. But he also meant to include all the needs we require to maintain a happy, healthy, and harmonious life.

In order to obtain our daily bread, all we have to do is claim it; we have to ask God for it and be aware that God provides all kinds of daily bread not just "to" us but "through" us. Let's take a closer look.

The source of daily bread

Cancer patients tend to think of their potential for healing as coming from certain sources. "My doctor is my only hope" is a very widely held belief. Others think, "I have to do it all by myself." Still other patients think diet, exercise, and prayer are the way.

The truth is each of these is merely a channel through which healing may come. It is God who is the source of all our daily bread, including healing and treatment. Believe it: The number of possible channels is infinite, but the source is One.

For the cancer patient, I believe this includes the possibility for the exact type of treatment you need at the exact time you need it. Face it: If you've been on the cancer journey for any length of time, the particular channel through which you are receiving treatment has very likely changed, perhaps more than once.

Cancer treatments come and go. Chemotherapy is notorious for initially shrinking tumors but then proving ineffective. Tumors develop resistance, and often there is no further response to the treatment.

Many in the oncology community still say, "The patient 'failed' chemotherapy." The truth is the chemotherapy failed, not the patient. But this is just one of many, many channels for treatment and healing.

For the cancer patient, "Give us this day our daily bread" means when one treatment door closes, others remain open. The mistake we make is to confuse a single channel with the single source, God. That misconception can lead us to think we have been abandoned without further supply.

Oh, that cancer patients would realize, through the hour-by-hour practice of the presence of God, that God is always their supply. Then they would see their current treatment as only one of many possible channels through which healing may come. Then, if there is a failure of that channel, they can find another. In fact these new channels may often be better in many ways.

Praying for our daily bread is a belief in, and dependence on, God's supply, our loving heavenly Father's supply. When we hold the conviction that God is our supply, and when we understand that God's supply does not fail, we can then affirm with confidence, "Thy will be done, Lord."

"I don't like what I heard you say," shared one

of our retreat participants, a man with advanced lung cancer. "I need more medical certainty. I need less divine dependency."

For the Christian going through cancer, dependence on the Lord is exactly what we need to be feeling. It doesn't mean we refuse conventional treatment, but it does mean we come to understand God as the source of all healing. And the moment we are not dependent is the moment we have backed away from truly living by faith.

Medical certainty? There is no such thing. Less divine dependency? That is a very dangerous, egotistical, and foolish idea.

Reliance on God as our source is our only hope. Then, when a healing channel fails, we can respond with comparative indifference, not panic and fear. We can look to God for all we need. Then the new channel, which is but a matter of detail, will present itself.

The presence of God

Praying "Give us this day our daily bread" also signifies the personal realization of the presence of God. This means that we live knowing God truly exists and is present with us here and now. He is not just a nominal presence but is the Great Reality, our living and breathing Bread of Life.

When you have the Bread of Life, you possess all things. Jesus called this level of experience "bread" because it is nourishment for our souls. It is exactly what Jesus was speaking of when he was tempted by Satan to command a stone to become a loaf of bread. Even though he was tired and hungry from his time in the wilderness, Jesus replied, "It is written, 'That man shall not live by bread alone' " (Luke 4:4). He was teaching us to develop and possess a spiritual strength that transcends hunger, illness, and even death.

Daily bread is here for you through the cancer journey. This means the actual experience of God's presence. More than merely thinking about God or talking about God, we can experience life through this miraculous daily presence. This, in the fullest sense, is what daily bread is all about, the thing that counts most. And our individual daily bread experience heals even when a cure may not be forthcoming.

Now healing is realized: First the healing of the spirit, then the healing of the mind, and finally the healing of the body. God is the One Source of it all.

Thank you, Lord, for giving us today our daily bread.

chapter

7

Our Father which art in heaven,
Hallowed be thy name.
Thy kingdom come.
Thy will be done in earth,
as it is in heaven.
Give us this day our daily bread.

And forgive us our debts,
as we forgive our debtors.

And lead us not into temptation,
but deliver us from evil:
For thine is the kingdom, and the power,
and the glory, for ever.

he Greatest Prayer now comes to a strategic crossroads.
We are brought to the issue of forgiveness, one of the
central challenges of the Christian walk.

Forgiveness saved my life

I hated my father, my earthly father. And I believed he
hated me. My recollections of youth are not pleasant.
I was constantly berated by my dad. I was called an
idiot, a lamebrain, a good-for-nothing, blankety-blank
disappointment.

In sports, in school, at home, at play, even in the
memorization of Bible verses, I was inadequate, and he
was there to emphatically point out my shortcomings.

It wasn't just the words my dad used—the biting
profanities—it was also his tone of voice and facial
expressions as he yelled.

With each word, there would be a pause, an accusing
intonation that seared into my consciousness. His face
had anger written all over it. I felt unloved, unworthy,
and more than once, I felt physically threatened. But only
once do I remember him slapping me hard, right across
the face with an open hand.

One Sunday afternoon, our family cleaned out some
junk from the garage. Our little village had a dump,
a junk pile on the outskirts of town where trash was
brought to be buried or burned.

We loaded up the back of the pickup, and just before we left, my father said, "I'll grab the shotgun. Let's see if we can get us a rat." I froze. I was perhaps 7 or 8 years old at the time, and in my mind, I believed my dad was taking me to the dump to kill me. My heart raced. I was certain my death was his intent. I was petrified.

After unloading the truck, Dad reached for the shotgun. I remember turning my back, thinking that I did not want to see that gun raised and pointed at me. As it turned out, he lined up some old bottles, and we each took a few turns at target practice. But the bone-chilling fear remained with me.

As I grew older and stronger, I stood taller than my father. I knew if I wanted to, I could physically overpower him. He knew it too, and the name-calling seemed to lessen.

But the emotional and psychological damage had been done. We seldom spoke. At best we coexisted with a thinly disguised contempt toward each other. I certainly hated him, and I believed he hated me.

When I was a teen, my father was committed to a mental institution for a period of time. The shame I felt in front of my friends and classmates was difficult to endure. The fact that a girlfriend broke up with me just reinforced my belief that I was inept and undeserving of any good.

It was my goal to leave home as soon as possible. I did so the summer after my high school graduation. I wanted to get as far away as possible from the abuses and perceived victimization I had suffered.

As a college student, I repeated the role and lapsed into victim behavior again and again. I went through periods of psychological pain, depression, and self-pity. Alcohol became my best friend, bringing temporary, hollow relief.

I discovered I had fallen into a trap. I was imprisoned by my own anger and the rage I felt against my father. Rather than protecting me from my past or any further pain, my hate now become my jailer. My hate was causing me to repeat my past.

It was not until cancer, nearly 20 years later, that I became aware of what I was doing to myself and those around me. Thankfully, my wife, Linda, was on a spiritual path. By her example, she pointed the way.

At one of the lowest points in my cancer journey, Linda helped me begin to understand how blaming both my earthly father and my heavenly Father, one for abuse and one for perceived abandonment, simply added to the suffering I was experiencing.

Forgiveness came into my consciousness at about this same time. From my deathbed, I was contacting people on the telephone, looking for survivors, wanting to learn from them what I might do to get well again.

Colleen, a survivor of metastatic breast cancer, was one of those people from whom I drew strength and encouragement. From our first phone conversation, Colleen asked me about forgiveness. She was convinced that forgiveness—the letting go and sincere release of anger and hurt—was something nearly all cancer patients who wished to survive were required to do.

After weeks of listening to her speak of forgiving, I began to realize this was central to my own journey to wellness. Colleen had done a great deal of forgiving. She shared with me that each day she felt greater freedom from the pain and anger associated with her past.

"And now, at 51 years of age," she said, "I am beginning to experience happiness and even moments of joy for the first time in my life."

Colleen had let go of the painful perceptions that imprisoned her. It became very clear; I needed to do the same.

Forgiveness as a way of life

A toxic relationship with parents, a spouse, coworkers, or significant others is a common characteristic among cancer patients. I ask you to examine this issue closely.

Of course this is exactly what Jesus was teaching the world when he said, "Forgive us our debts, as we forgive our debtors." Note the condition: We are forgiven as we forgive. Jesus drafted this declaration in such a way that we are forced to confront our own need to forgive others before we can receive forgiveness.

There is simply no escape; we must positively and definitely extend forgiveness to everyone to whom we owe forgiveness. Jesus leaves no wiggle room on this issue. He constructed the Greatest Prayer to intentionally draw our mind and spirit to the fact that we are obliged to forgive our enemies, with complete sincerity, or never again recite the Lord's Prayer.

Forgive us as we forgive others. It's there. There's no dispute. Jesus said it. Forgiveness starts with you and me.

It is critical to evaluate and resolve this issue of harboring hostility and resentment, especially for cancer patients. The good news is you can do this work even if the person in the dispute is dead. Furthermore, you can do this work whether or not you are in contact with the person.

The frightening and yet utterly exhilarating truth is the focus of forgiveness is on you, on your release, on your letting go. You are changing your own perceptions and beliefs and the feelings they create.

Many cancer patients do not want to forgive. That was certainly me. After years of trying denial as my chief coping mechanism, deep down I did not want to forgive my father because I felt so wronged. I felt that to forgive him would be the same as condoning the cruelty and injustice I had experienced. But then Linda's wisdom and positive faith came to my aid. "Failing to forgive," she shared, "is like holding a burning coal in the palm of your hand. The only person you are hurting is you."

Maybe it was that image of a coal burning the palm of my hand. Ouch! It made the point. My unwillingness to forgive was hurting only me.

One important perspective for changing your beliefs and attitudes, one that is of immense help in the work of forgiveness, is the insight that we all do the best we can with the level of understanding we have at the time. We can use this knowledge to forgive those who have caused us harm. And, perhaps even more important, we can use this tool to forgive ourselves.

My father really didn't know any better. He came from a large family where he was the youngest and the smallest. They were farmers, and his father was an abusive alcoholic. My dad modeled in his own family what he had experienced in the family of his youth. He was doing his best, given his level of understanding.

Once I understood and accepted my father's limited relationship abilities, there was a change. No big reconciliation took place between us. Yet the shift in my attitude brought about real change for me.

Forgive us as we forgive others. This is God's plan for forgiveness, an insight for his most cherished children. Forgive and you'll be forgiven.

I'll admit, it took some real effort on my part. And there was a part of me that still wanted to hold on to a piece of that rage. But finally, with integrity, I could say that I forgave my dad, that I totally released and let go of those toxic emotions, and that I wished him every good thing.

Perhaps you have a difficult relationship you need to release through forgiveness. I ask you to meditate on the turning point of the Lord's Prayer: "Forgive us our debts, as we forgive our debtors."

With our release of forgiveness, we release God's power to accomplish his will through these seemingly impossible situations.

It is very possible to acknowledge your hurt, live with it, and still forgive. You can be a forgiver even when a relationship continues to be difficult.

A breast cancer patient who was a regular at our "Lunch Bunch" support group had a poor relationship with her mother, who was always critical and negative. After our friend was diagnosed, her mother's telephone calls and visits were filled with gloom and doom. She clearly believed her daughter was going to die, and soon.

Once the daughter had the realization that her mother was doing the best she could with the level of understanding she had, the daughter could extend forgiveness. But she also recognized she had the right to refuse her mother's messages. The woman told her mother that she would be in touch when she wanted to talk, but otherwise she could not take her mother's calls while she was in the middle of her healing work.

Now, nearly nine years later, she is free of disease and once again in communication with her mother.

Forgive. Be forgiven. I call Jesus' instruction on forgiveness a true miracle generator. If you are a cancer patient and seeking God's blessing in your life, this is the course to take—Cancer Survival 101.

It's all right there for us. We are to declare that we have actually and sincerely forgiven, and forgiven all—anyone who we perceive may have wronged us. It's our own release, our personal letting go we are after. And Jesus makes our personal claim on divine forgiveness dependent upon that act. Forgiveness then becomes our way of life. I couldn't recommend more highly living life as a continuous exercise in forgiveness.

Forgiveness: a power surge

Dear people who are struggling with cancer, I cannot emphasize this point enough. There are very few people in the world who have not at some time or another been hurt, deeply hurt, or disappointed or rejected or deceived or injured or misled by someone else. These experiences stay with us, haunting our memories and usually festering or becoming open emotional and spiritual wounds. There is just one remedy. The one and only way to heal them is by forgiveness.

Tragic as it may be, few people on the spiritual path practice complete forgiveness. Many people acknowledge a general forgiveness. That's easy. Almost anyone can rise above the thought of resentment for a trifling loss and offer forgiveness in a general sense.

Forgiving us our debts as we forgive our debtors requires us not only to forgive the trifles and forgive in general but also to forgive the deepest hurts and most horrific acts that seem all but impossible to do.

We worked with a woman in California who was repeatedly raped by her father and brother during her teenage years. I can remember her despair when she said, "It's too much to ask. It's so painful. It's impossible. I simply cannot forgive them."

But the Lord's Prayer makes our own forgiveness come from God and our escape from pain and suffering dependent on this very act. There is no other way to interpret this teaching. No matter how deeply we might have been hurt or how terribly we might have suffered, forgiveness must be done.

When we forgive completely, I am convinced that God's supernatural power surges through our lives. When we extend forgiveness, we see God's mighty presence. We also see tremendous results that can only be explained as coming from the hand of God.

I not only had my father to forgive, but I had a whole list of people to work through. These included others in my family and close friends as well as neighbors and business acquaintances.

What strikes me about forgiveness is how simple it is to extend and how difficult it is to sincerely mean. This was my experience with my coworker Ollie, one of my most troublesome relationships to resolve.

I employed a simple three-step process that is widely used to forgive.

First, you call the person's name and image to mind. So I would bring Ollie to mind.

Second, you forgive and release out loud. "Ollie," I said, "I forgive you. I release you."

Third, you affirm God's goodness in their lives as you bless them. "Ollie, I wish you God's every blessing."

The tricky part is to complete each of the three steps with utter and complete sincerity. Anything short of that is a sham. You must hold yourself accountable for being sincere at every step.

So I went down my list of people I had to forgive.

There was my father—and then Ollie. There was my mother—and then Ollie. There was an old girlfriend—and then Ollie. I kept coming back to Ollie. I could not release him and bless him and be sincere about it.

My forgiveness efforts continued for nearly a week. Finally I called Ollie and made an appointment to see him. And in one of the most difficult things I have ever done, I stood face-to-face with a person I resented and said, "I forgive you. I release you, Ollie. I want only God's richest blessings in your life."

Wow! That was tough.

I left Ollie's house a free man. I was able to say, "I'm free! I'm free! I'm free!"

How did God honor this act of forgiveness? I can trace the exact turning point in my physical recovery to that moment of forgiveness. And today I do my utmost to make forgiveness my way of life.

Willingness to forgive

Are you receptive to this point? I hope and pray you are. The concept of forgiveness starts with your receptivity. More fundamental than any three-step process, the essential issue is your willingness to forgive. If you simply and sincerely desire to set your offender free, the greater part of your work is done.

Setting others free is setting yourself free. When

you hold hostility against anyone, you are bound to that person through the rope of your hate. The very person whom you dislike most in the world is the very person to whom you are attaching yourself.

Remember, your thoughts will, at some point, be drawn into your life. Is that what you seek? Is that the way you wish to live? Could lack of forgiveness be a contributing factor in your illness?

When we ordinary followers of Jesus extend forgiveness, we are filled with a grace and power that transcend our hostile thoughts of resentment, remorse, and recrimination.

The "hand of the Lord" is a biblical term for the power and presence of God in the lives of his people. Forgiveness brings, I believe, the Lord's hand to your life.

Does this mean we must achieve reconciliation? Does forgiveness require us to like our offender?

I think not. We are not required to like that person. But we are required to love him or her. We are not required to totally reconcile with that person. But we are required to live at peace with that person. It means living out the Christmas announcement, "On Earth, peace, good will toward men."

I also believe you don't need to keep repeating your sincere forgiveness. In the future, whenever the memory of the offender comes to mind, bless him or her and release the thought. After a short period of time, you will find the bitterness and resentment have disappeared. You're free!

Suddenly, as I write this, I want to fall on my knees in prayerful forgiveness. Join me.

When was the last time you took a searching personal inventory to determine if hostility could be poisoning a corner of your heart?

When was the last time you fully released a grudge you are holding against your spouse or coworker?

When was the last time you fervently prayed for your perceived enemy, "I wish you God's greatest blessings"?

Forgive us our debts, as we forgive our debtors. Healing, true healing, does not happen without it.

chapter

8

Our Father which art in heaven,
Hallowed be thy name.
Thy kingdom come.
Thy will be done in earth,
as it is in heaven.
Give us this day our daily bread.
And forgive us our debts,
as we forgive our debtors.

*And lead us not into temptation,
but deliver us from evil.*

For thine is the kingdom, and the power,
and the glory, for ever.

A stumbling block causes people to trip, to lose their balance, perhaps even to fall. This clause in the Lord's Prayer is a stumbling block for millions of believers.

Think about it. How could a good God lead anyone into temptation? Why would we ever consider that a loving Heavenly Father might allow his child to come close to circumstances that are evil?

I believe that Jesus, in teaching us the Greatest Prayer, inserted this clause to remind us to pray for guidance and deliverance from any spiritual test that may be too much for us. And in a real sense, cancer is one of those tests.

Spiritual awareness

Christians on a healing journey are, we hope, becoming more self-aware. We become increasingly aware of our human limits, frailties, and weaknesses. And perhaps most critical, spiritual seekers grow keenly aware of the personal need for absolute dependence on our Heavenly Father for everything—literally everything, even the next breath we draw.

It's another required course of instruction, Spiritual Fitness 101, whose learning outcome is the realization that we need to live every moment in and through God. That awareness is the gateway to healing.

It is not long before our increasing spiritual

self-awareness begins to make clear the myriad of temptations and evils that surround us. We now look in the mirror and see what lies behind our own eyes. We begin to see that living a life on the spiritual path requires a consistency between what we believe, how we think, the way we feel, and what we do. It's a purity of intention followed by a consistency of action that we seek. And this, to the spiritually self-aware, is no small challenge.

At this point, the Lord's Prayer gives us great hope. In a real sense, the true inner meaning of the entire prayer is a short course in personal spiritual growth. The journey through cancer can be the teacher, provided we students become aware of our dependence on our Heavenly Father.

A sensitive heart

Jesus knew full well the perils and difficulties that are presented to us as we walk the spiritual path. The more time we spend in prayer and meditation, the more sensitive we become. In fact, if we truly begin to achieve a degree of spiritual maturity, we will become acutely sensitive to our own state of being as well as that of the world around us.

For most people, that more sensitive heart seems to be a desirable outcome. But that sensitive heart yields an awareness of temptations, even circumstances of evil that escape the radar screen of the people who are not as spiritually aware.

For example, what many believe to be just good fun may now become an issue of moral failure for the person gaining spiritual self-awareness.

I am clearly guilty. I might see a woman who is looking good—great posture, stylish clothes, and a big smile. My first thought is, "Doesn't she look great? I'd like to meet her."

Then, in the middle of an animated conversation, I catch myself sneaking a glance at her figure—a millisecond scan of her body. And if I am not careful, in my mind I go from enjoying the conversation to admiring her body.

To some, that might be a minor transgression. To me, it is no ordinary fault. It's lust, and God is not going to bless lust. If I find myself in that situation, I do my best to stir up my spiritual power and say, "Lord, help. Let me be your representative here, now."

That's spiritual awareness. I am typically not tempted to steal or lie or kill as the world defines it. But I realize my thoughts, words, and behavior may "steal" hope from someone. Or being less than forthcoming may result in a "lie" of omission. Or that wishing people ill will could be the equivalent of "killing" their spirit.

Spiritual awareness requires higher standards.

Jesus knew about these trials, temptations, and difficulties. He knew that if we are to grow stronger spiritual muscles, we have to have trials to overcome. He also knew those trials and temptations should not be greater than what our current level of spiritual understanding could resist and overcome.

Wrong attitudes, faulty motives, toxic emotions, self-reliance, pride, and more—they all await us on the spiritual pathway. That is why Jesus taught, "Lead us not ... Deliver us from ...."

But odd as it may seem, trials and temptations can actually be of benefit to us. In fact, you can and should expect them. Now that you're in the middle of the cancer journey, you have one big trial. It is going to leave you, emotionally and spiritually, in one of two ways: bitter or better.

Soon after you step onto this spiritual path and make this walk your primary strategy to conquer cancer, you will experience moments that seem overwhelming. Though these are grand opportunities for spiritual growth, lurking in the corner of your mind is the thought that you have remained as small and as weak as ever.

From your human perspective, cancer is certainly not a mountaintop moment. But from a spiritual perspective, it has enormous promise.

It's because God can use cancer to refine you spiritually, to cleanse, purify, and raise you to new levels of spiritual power. Perhaps cancer is, in part, God's way of molding you into the person he wants you to be.

And if, in these moments, we learn to align with God and be open to change and to correct areas that he brings to light, then we will pass the test. We will develop new levels of spiritual fitness. And I believe we will be spiritually rewarded.

Cancer: a test of faith

That was certainly my case. As I continued to physically decline, losing weight, being confined to bed, and taking morphine to control the pain, I prayed constantly. I prayed by simply putting myself in the presence of God and then listening. This, I believe, is the doorway to spiritual self-awareness.

It soon became clear to me that God was more interested in changing and healing me than he was in changing or healing my cancer. It was I who needed work before he could deal with the illness.

I was tempted to slip into moments of self-pity and the evil of despair. But then, in the quiet of the presence of God, I would pray, "Oh, Lord, lead me not into the temptation of self-pity. Heavenly Father, deliver me from the evil of despair."

I believe God was testing me in areas where I was weakest, where I needed most to grow spiritually. You've probably found the same thing. It's natural to feel overwhelmed in the area of your greatest vulnerability.

I used to have a serious jealousy streak. It seemed that everyone I met had better or more material possessions than I. Whether it was houses or cars or investment portfolios, they had them and I didn't. I ended up envious, bitter, and jealous.

It was a spiritual test that took me years to finally pass. Today I can honestly rejoice at the good fortune of others. I can see it as a blessing, as proof that God rewards those who seek him.

On your cancer journey, you can expect moments of weakness. But remember that even in the midst of your need, you can find spiritual strength. Then you'll pass the spiritual test of cancer.

I pray you receive this truth with an open heart, because none of us is beyond testing and learning. I recently counseled one of America's most prominent pastors, who was going through a life-threatening illness. Near the end of our talk he said, "I don't think this is a spiritual test for me. I constantly examine myself. I stand pure before my Lord."

The test of spiritual pride stands above all other challenges. Spiritual superiority and self-righteousness are perhaps the most deadly of all attitudes. We all fare best when we humble ourselves before God. Even the most advanced student, like this pastor, has much to learn.

I pray that God will lead you away from the temptation of hopelessness and deliver you from the evil of despair. I pray that you will see the spiritual side of cancer as God's way of asking you to examine your character, his attempt to refine you, and his way of drawing you closer to him.

Summon strength for today and faith for tomorrow. Pray "Lead us not into temptation, but deliver us from evil." You'll be amazed at the healing that is in store for you.

chapter

9

Our Father which art in heaven,
Hallowed be thy name.
Thy kingdom come.
Thy will be done in earth,
as it is in heaven.
Give us this day our daily bread.
And forgive us our debts,
as we forgive our debtors.
And lead us not into temptation,
but deliver us from evil:

For thine is the kingdom, and the power, and the glory, for ever.

*C*ancer is an unparalleled opportunity for spiritual growth. Provided we are open to its lessons, working daily for understanding and guidance from the Holy Spirit, we will never find ourselves stranded in a place of spiritual abandonment. God is with us even in the darkest moments of pain, nausea, hair loss, and the myriad of dehumanizing experiences of the cancer journey.

Then, with certainty, we can say, "Father, 'thine is the kingdom, and the power, and the glory, for ever.'" This is an affirmation that both comforts and heals.

This clause of the Lord's Prayer is all about the omnipotence and eternal omnipresence of God. I believe it is especially, vividly about that presence through the darkness of cancer.

The sentence "For thine is the kingdom, and the power, and the glory, for ever" does not appear in all translations of Matthew nor in Luke's account of the Lord's Prayer. Its exact origin is unclear. A similar Old Testament version appears in 1 Chronicles 29. We know it came to us through the early Christian church and tradition has kept it alive. It's a wonderful affirmation.

The affirmation's essential truth is that God is not only everywhere but is also everything, the source of all life and power, all existing to bring expression to God's omnipotence, forever.

The "kingdom" is referring to all creation, on every level. It certainly means physical creations of this world and beyond, plus the inner emotional and spiritual capacity we possess and can develop.

The "power" refers to God's power. It is an acknowledgment that we have limited human power but unlimited divine power available to us. For the cancer patient, it is a reminder to rely not on man's ability but on God's ability as our source for healing.

Of course, the "glory" is linked to God's radiance, splendor, and majesty. It is also an affirmation of God's glorious demonstrations in every area of our lives. For the cancer patient, this is the demonstration of healing. This means God's kingdom, in all its glory, is here for us, now, in some form of healing. Through that healing we share in God's glory, even though we are clearly not that glory.

A publisher sent me a manuscript, looking for my endorsement for a soon-to-be-published work. It included a full-page magazine ad depicting a woman, full of pride and anger, wagging her finger directly in the face of her doctor. The caption read: "Sometimes you just want to scream, 'Listen, you dummy!'" The book was entitled *I Can Heal Myself.* I declined to write an endorsement.

We can't heal ourselves. Even though we have been given countless self-healing capabilities, we are not the power behind the healing. And please understand, our doctors can't heal. They can treat cancer, removing the problem or causing it to be chemically or biologically altered so that it is no longer life-threatening. But that is not healing.

Recall our definition of healing. It is a wholeness, a soundness, a peacefulness, a complete integration of body, mind, and spirit founded upon the teachings and the living example of Jesus Christ. For the Christian, healing is not a medical fix but a way of life. God is the only source of healing. And only God deserves the glory that surrounds our healing.

Yes, you should choose diet and exercise routines that contribute to greater health. Yes, your doctor can cut, poison, and burn the bad cells. Yes, I clearly understand, those things have a place. But none heal.

God alone does the healing. Humanly speaking, we just can't do it. God heals. And it's all done for God's glory.

Giving your heavenly Father the credit and glory for your healing is required. It must become our primary motive. We can give this glory to God by:
- Growing spiritually through the study of His Word.
- Praying earnestly for his will to be done in and through us.
- Worshiping out of love and gratitude, not duty.

- Being more Christ-like in character.
- Loving others without conditions, as Jesus loved.
- Serving with our God-given talents to benefit others.
- Witnessing by showing others the way through our example.

All are important. I ask you to make them central to your life. But one stands out. I personally believe our living witness is the most powerful way to give glory to God.

A matter of motives

Our healing is greatly influenced by our motives. Our motives are the set of the sails of our heart. These sails need to be lifted high in order to bring glory to God. One sure way to do this is to trust God—no matter what. It means deeply trusting in the Greatest Prayer's affirmation, "Thine is the kingdom, and the power, and the glory, for ever."

The most powerful living witness of trusting God that I know is a very special woman, Lois Ware. She exemplifies triumph over tragedy. She also deeply trusts that her life's miraculous journey is all a demonstration of God's glory.

Lois' "challenges," as she calls them, started early. In high school she was involved in three auto accidents, a train wreck, and a school bus accident and was nearly asphyxiated by carbon monoxide.

Following her marriage, Lois became violently ill during her second pregnancy. Test after test provided no answers. Finally a nephrologist diagnosed a rare kidney disease and recommended complete removal of the damaged kidney, a procedure never before attempted for this illness in a late pregnancy. Doctors feared for the lives of both mother and child.

"I refused to accept that fear and hopelessness," said Lois. "Six and a half months pregnant, I went ahead with the surgery. With God's help, I was determined we would both survive." They did. And Lois' case was written up as a first-of-a-kind in the medical literature. People everywhere called it a miracle.

Lois and her husband decided to leave her Midwest roots for the promises of California. She found a job in the booming real estate business and became active in a positive, Bible-based church. It was just what she needed.

"Life was good," Lois said. "I constantly thanked God for miracle after miracle."

But then, more challenges. Lois was diagnosed with a blood clot in her brain. Soon after, she suffered a stroke. Thankfully, it did not leave her impaired. A tumor was discovered in her right leg. Initially the only treatment was thought to be amputation, but surgery successfully removed only the tumor, which proved to be benign.

"Another set of miracles," Lois said. "God is so good."

The Ware family was an active one, and one of their favorite sports was cycling. They rode bicycles all over the Western United States, often doing "century rides" of 100 miles at a time. They were very fit.

One Saturday, halfway through such a ride along the Pacific Coast Highway, Lois was struck by a truck pulling a trailer. The force of the blow knocked Lois down and pulled her under the truck, and she was run over by the rear wheels of both the truck and trailer. As the hit-and-run driver sped away, Lois lay unconscious in a growing pool of blood on Highway 1 just north of San Diego.

The group with whom she was riding called for an emergency unit and the police. Lois was airlifted to the nearest trauma unit. Not expected to live, Lois had a badly mangled foot; multiple broken bones including her hand, pelvis, and nose; and massive internal injuries and blood loss. She had landed on her face and more than 300 stitches were required to stop the bleeding. "Oh, Lord," pleaded her husband, Russ, "please save her."

Days later, slowly, painfully, she regained consciousness. Her mangled foot was the most troublesome injury. A team of orthopedic surgeons delivered the diagnosis.

"Your foot is crushed beyond repair," said one of the surgeons. "We can't operate. All we can do is put it in a cast. The rest is in God's hands."

"In God's hands. That's a good place to put it," Lois told them.

"OK, but you'll never walk on your own again," said one surgeon.

"You watch," Lois responded. "If this is in God's hands, I will walk."

Through a long and difficult time of recovery, Lois kept saying and believing, "God is going to use this for his glory." "God has a plan for me, a plan for good." "The Lord is the strength of my life; of whom shall I be afraid?"

Friends came to Lois' hospital room and literally surrounded her with care and love. Impromptu prayer services were held. She constantly thanked her doctors and caregivers. And, of course, she shared with others about her very real relationship with Jesus Christ and God.

"Believers, believe!" Lois declared. "I believe God's promises. I trust God and believe that he is in charge. I believe I will get through this, and I plan to live a long life. What's the worst that could happen? Death? Then I would be with Jesus. That's not so bad. That's my ultimate goal anyway!"

Lois Ware's stellar example of a deeply trusting spirit is exceedingly powerful. It's an example for all of us. In more than 20 years of witnessing healings, I believe this set of the sails of one's heart is the difference between life and death.

Lois' trust in God is what makes her such a great heroine of the faith, a true believer, and God's walking miracle among us. We have much to learn from people like Lois and their stories.

Through month after month of intense rehabilitation, Lois began to regain her mobility. Every day she would affirm, "With God's help, I will walk!"

"Inch by inch, anything's a cinch," Lois declared. First a wheelchair, then a walker, followed by crutches and bulky orthopedic braces. "These braces are real fashion trendsetters," Lois would say with a laugh. Finally, after an arduous journey, she was able to walk with a slight limp that eventually disappeared. Lois was certain her troubles were behind her.

"Thank you, God," she prayed. "Thank you, Lord, for another miracle."

But Lois would soon need yet another miracle. Just three days after discarding her crutches, she was incapacitated by severe abdominal pains. Her physician noticed what seemed to be an enlarged lymph node and recommended a biopsy as soon as possible.

The supreme test

Lois had arrived in the territory held up for examination in the book of Job. She was suffering—again. The age-old question had to be asked: Why do bad things happen to good people?

The biopsy revealed a malignant, non-Hodgkins lymphoma. Though Lois was still recovering from her near-fatal bicycle accident, she began chemotherapy treatments for cancer.

I believe there are times when evil surrounds us. Many times, I believe evil is visited most upon people who are becoming the greatest good for the Lord. In fact, the more we glorify God, the more we should be prepared to confront spiritual attack. This may be your experience also.

This was certainly Lois' journey. She began the difficult cancer treatments, determined she would not get sick or lose her hair. Her medical team laughed at her attitude. "This stuff makes you very sick," they said. "And you're going to lose *all* your hair."

Lois' faith never wavered. Although she did lose her hair, she never did get sick. And all the while Lois affirmed, "I trust God. He will use this cancer for good. I put it all into his hands. It's all going to demonstrate God's power and glory."

I ask you to stop for a moment and examine your own heart. Trusting God works miracles. This is not some passive, fatalistic trust. We speak here of an active faith, a deep trust, a living and breathing reliance on the character, strength, ability, and truth of the promises of Jesus Christ. It is through this trust that we can demonstrate God's kingdom, power, and glory in our lives, now and forever.

Do you have that same trust? Are your motives for seeking healing to demonstrate God's power and glory? Might there be room for ever-increasing spiritual growth in your life?

I have been ministering to people going through cancer for more than 20 years. The single major spiritual insight from two decades of this work is this: God is more interested in changing your heart than he is in eliminating your illness. His all-powerful presence is waiting to see changed motives. When that happens, healing of all kinds will appear.

Perhaps you are in the middle of your own cancer battle right now. And you're doing what I first did. You're praying, "Lord, take this cancer away." You're asking God, "Deliver me from evil."

That is a legitimate prayer. I hope "cancer free" is your personal experience. But maybe you're missing the point of why you were given the gift of this exceedingly difficult experience. Like Lois, it could be that God is trying to do a greater work in you. He's molding and changing your heart. He's deepening your faith.

But maybe you are so busy trying to fight the cancer that the work God is attempting to do cannot be done.

You may be so focused on the poor statistics and the difficult treatments and the paralyzing fear that you haven't taken the time to look within, to listen for the healing that God may be attempting to bring you.

I recently asked Lois what she would have other cancer patients know. She wrote, "Trust God. Don't complicate healing. Trust.

"The most frightening time," she continued, "is the dark of night when everyone's asleep, and you find yourself awake, seemingly alone, with your fears and worries. In those moments, I ask every cancer patient to relax and give yourself completely to God—His kingdom, and trust God for healing—His power, and thank God for all—His glory, forever and ever.

"Secure in this knowledge, we can fall asleep knowing that God will always have the last word. And it will be good, no matter what."

Thank you, Lois Ware—a trusting heart that reflects God's kingdom, power, and glory, this moment and forever.

That is not only healing for cancer, but it is also healing for life.

*Making the Greatest
Prayer Yours*

J challenge you to make the Lord's Prayer the foundation of your journey through cancer. Weave its power into the very fabric of your everyday life. To do this, I encourage you to follow the simple plan outlined here for the next 40 days. I promise you, it will transform your health and your life.

Why 40 days? In the Bible, when God wanted to prepare someone for something special, it often took 40 days. That was true of Noah, Moses, and David. But I think it was most significant when Jesus spent 40 days in the wilderness. He prayed. He came out empowered.

Think of your cancer as your spiritual wilderness. Pray. Then during the next 40 days, I believe you will be empowered.

An invitation

I ask you to make a personal commitment to join me each and every day for the next 40 days to:

1. Pray the Lord's Prayer every morning. Keep a record of your daily prayer time by marking it off on a calendar.

2. In your own handwriting, write out the Lord's Prayer on a card, making this prayer your own. Keep the card visible in a place where you will be reminded of your new vision.

3. Reread this little book once a week during the

"Are you trying to do too much? Shouldn't you rest more often?" Her care and concern were central to my getting well again.

But my health did not deteriorate; it started to improve. The more I dedicated myself to living in the presence of God, to praying and doing, the stronger I felt physically and emotionally.

Some people said, "Greg, it's a miracle!" I agree. It was and is a miracle, but not in the dramatic sense that many people expect. It was a miracle that is still unfolding. And my health—now more than two decades since I was told I had 30 days to live—remains strong and is but one aspect of the miracle.

I am convinced one of the reasons I remain alive is that God is not done with me yet. There are things he would do through me provided I remain in the role of his servant. Today the little organization Linda and I started has expanded around the world. We are in five countries and serve a host of third-world countries. The books and supporting materials have also been translated into 29 different languages.

I do not share this to impress you. I share it as a testimony that God can take an imperfect person with a sincere heart and work miracles in his or her health and life and in the world.

I hope for something very similar for you.

Pray the Lord's Prayer. See it as your open invitation to God that says, "Use me. Use this cancer experience. Here I am, Lord. Send me."

God always answers that kind of prayer. The answer will often take you by surprise. You may think you know what you want from God, but God often has other ideas. This prayer can be a real learning experience, teaching you to stretch your faith muscles. You will often come to new understandings of God, of others, and of yourself with a clarity that you would never have experienced before you dropped to your knees and uttered the Greatest Prayer. Pray with me for the next 40 days:

Our Father which art in heaven,
Hallowed be thy name.
Thy kingdom come,
Thy will be done in earth,
as it is in heaven.
Give us this day our daily bread.
And forgive us our debts,
as we forgive our debtors.
And lead us not into temptation,
but deliver us from evil:
For thine is the kingdom, and the power,
and the glory, for ever.

I've seen some amazing things happen in the lives

and health of cancer patients who prayed, who grabbed the hem of God's garment and did not let go.

I think of it as the glory of a perfect sunrise. Prayer pierces the darkness of despair with a ray of light. The possibility of hope infuses and warms the spirit. Spiritual expectations shift. The prayers become more courageous, more faith filled. Healing is seen in a fuller, more complete light. And the person knows a growing excitement and anticipation of what God has next in store. A much brighter tomorrow—physically, emotionally, and spiritually—is the happy result.

I trust you have now found the amazing power and truth in the Lord's Prayer. Praying "Our Father, your will be done … here and now, in my life" always brings healing on many different levels. I hope you can begin to see changes already.

Make this prayer a regular, meaningful, and vital part of your life. It will be a new life. The wondrous changes you realize as you live in the presence of God will transform every phase of your being.

You'll see your doubt turned to faith, despair turned to hope, and fear turned to love.

It all results in a glorious legacy, now and hereafter. And in the process, you will have conquered cancer.

I wish you well.

Resources to help you

Cancer Recovery Foundation is an award-winning ecumenical, faith-based, nonprofit organization whose mission is to help all people prevent and survive cancer.

The Foundation's Faith & Health Initiative reaches out to help in the following ways:

- Educate people about their cancer diagnosis and understand all their treatment options;

- Empower patients and family members to understand and mobilize their God-given healing capacity; and

- Encourage all people to employ faith and hope through the cancer experience.

For complete information on the variety of resources available, please visit:

www.CancerRecovery.org
In North America call
(800) 238-6479

Other books by Greg Anderson

The Cancer Conqueror

The Cancer Conqueror with Bible Study Guide
with Michael Gingerich

The Triumphant Patient

Cancer: 50 Essential Things to Do

Healing Wisdom

The 22 (Non-Negotiable) Laws of Wellness

Journeys with the Cancer Conqueror

Living Life on Purpose

Come, Let's Change the World
with George M. Leader